Stroke Recovery

How I Kick-Started My Stalled Stroke Recovery

I

Other books by this author

- **Microscopic Colitis**
- **Understanding Microscopic Colitis**
- **Vitamin D and Autoimmune Disease**
- **8 Ways to Prevent Pancreatic Cancer**
- **Why Magnesium Is the Key to Long-Term Health**

Stroke Recovery

How I Kick-Started My Stalled Stroke Recovery

Wayne Persky

Persky Farms

United States

First published and distributed in the United States of America
by:
Persky Farms, 19242 Darrs Creek Rd, Bartlett, TX 76511-4460. Tel.: (1)254-718-1125; Fa:
(1)254-527-3682. www.perskyfarms.com

Disclaimer and Legal Notice: The information contained in this book is intended sole▌
for general educational purposes, and is not intended, nor implied, to be a substitute f▊
professional medical advice relative to any specific medical condition or question. The
advice of a physician or other health care provider should always be sought for any que
tions regarding any medical condition. Specific diagnoses and therapies can only be
provided by the reader's physician. Any use of the information in this book is at the rea
er's discretion. The author and the publisher specifically disclaim any and all liability
arising directly or indirectly from the use or application of any information contained i▊
this book.

Please note that much of the information in this book is based on personal experience
and anecdotal evidence. Although the author and publisher have made every reasonab▊
attempt to achieve complete accuracy of the content, they assume no responsibility for
errors or omissions. If you should choose to use any of this information, use it accordin
to your best judgment, and at your own risk. Because your particular situation will no▊
exactly match the examples upon which this information is based, you should adjust
your use of the information and recommendations to fit your own personal situation.

This book does not recommend or endorse any specific tests, products, procedures, opi▊
ions, or other information that may be mentioned anywhere in the book. This informa
tion is provided for educational purposes, and reliance on any tests, products, procedures, or opinions mentioned in the book is solely at the reader's own risk.

Any trademarks, service marks, product names, or named features are assumed to be th
property of their respective owners, and are used only for reference. There is no implie▊
endorsement when these terms are used in this book.

ISBN 978-1-7328220-6-1

Table of Contents

Chapter 1

My Stroke and My Initial Recovery

A stroke will grab your undivided attention as soon as you realize what's happening to your body. When a stroke begins, we have no way of knowing how far it will proceed, or how severely it's going to affect our body, until the destruction is over. Since it's normal to fear the unknown, and things that we don't understand, fear is almost surely going to dominate our thinking, once we recognize that we're having a stroke. And fear can make it difficult to make decisions, but if nothing else, it should prompt us to get to the emergency room of the nearest hospital as quickly as possible. Once we get to the ER, our fate will be in the hands of someone who is trained to deal with strokes, and hopefully, he or she will make the right decisions.

Assuming that we survive the initial stroke, we will experience two basic outcomes.

1. 1. There will be damage to our neurological system.

2. 2. Our brain and our body will try to recover, afterward.

Stroke Recovery

It may appear that a lot of muscle damage has also occurred. But this is an aberration, caused by the loss of muscle control due to nerve damage. The actual damage is basically all neurological. But unless a proper physical rehabilitation program is promptly initiated, those muscles will atrophy rather quickly, due to lack of use.

There's not much we can do about the first item on that short list, except to take an aspirin, and hope and pray for the best, as we call 911, or otherwise make arrangements to get to an emergency room as quickly as is reasonably possible (assuming that we're capable of doing that). But how well we're able to take advantage of the second item, depends on a lot of things. We may choose to let our doctors decide how we should approach recovery, and follow their advice to the letter. They're going to base their recommendations on whatever the currently-accepted medical policies of the hospital dictate as the best method for treating most stroke patients. Stroke recovery treatments have come a long way in recent years.

Or we could choose to just listen to our body, and let it dictate our course of action (or inaction). A better option is to try to maximize our recovery by following the advice of our doctors and using the medical approach, while supplementing that treatment with one or more alternative treatments that have been shown to be beneficial for improving stroke recovery. After all, more and more people are discovering every day that in some situations, the medical approach to certain healthcare issues can leave a lot to be desired. The medical approach relies on published research data providing proof of concept, before a treatment will be accepted. Because of that requirement, medical treatments are always a step or two behind new developments. That usually means that recommended treatments are several years behind technology. In some situations, alternative treatments may provide many benefits, with little added risk, or expense. Whatever we choose to do, how we decide to proceed can be extremely important for our future quality of life, because time is of the essence following a stroke. There is no proven limit to how long the body will try to recover. It's theoretically possible to make recovery progress for years, maybe even decades. And we probably all have our own individual maximum recovery potential. But there's no question that the greatest recovery potential exists during the first few weeks after a stroke, and it slowly diminishes as time passes.

Following a stroke, it may be days before we can even determine the total extent of the damage. But as we begin our recovery, how well we recover will depend on many factors, not the least of which is our attitude in general, and our degree of hope in particular. This is because, as we shall see later, a negative attitude and lack of hope leads to post-stroke depression. And arguably the worst effect of that depression may be to severely suppress our body's built-in attempts to recover. If the body doesn't (or can't) attempt to recover, then recovery may become impossible Because our best potential for recovery is available early-on, obviously, the faster we can recover, the better off we'll be. After a few months, recovery will become progressively slower.

Stroke Recovery

I'm not a medical professional (my formal education is in engineering and mathematics), but based on my own recovery, I believe that the harder we push ourselves (within reason), the more complete our recovery will be. That's sort of self-evident when we consider that recovering from a stroke requires relearning how to do so many things. We learn by repetition, so we have to practice if we want to become proficient at regaining control of our brains and our muscles. We will have some degree of recovery, even if we do nothing but rest all day and night. But we will recover faster and more completely, if we push ourselves to try to relearn how to regain the brainpower and muscle function that we've lost. Obviously, many stroke victims will face much more difficult issues than others, so we have to consider our limitations, as we go forward. And we have to remember that our bodies also need plenty of rest, to facilitate healing. Our bodies are designed so that our muscles and our brains heal while we're sleeping. That implies that without good sleep, both healing and learning will be compromised. But we have to expedite the learning process by exercising our brains and our muscles while we're awake.

Information is stored in our brains as we sleep, but that information must be loaded into the queue, so to speak, while we're awake. We load potential memory material by reading and/or thinking about that material. And we load muscle responses required to perform certain tasks into the queue by doing those tasks (or attempting to do them, if the stroke has left us unable to do them). Then those memories, and the ability to perform those tasks more capably, will be stored in our brains as we sleep.

My Stroke and My Initial Recovery

As we all know, strokes can have various specific causes, and the resulting physical and mental consequences tend to vary significantly. Medical experts warn us about the signs we should look for. Signs such as:

- Sudden numbness or weakness of muscles in our face, arm, or leg, especially if it occurs on one side of our body.
- Sudden confusion, or trouble speaking, or understanding what someone else is saying.
- Sudden trouble with our vision in one or both eyes.
- Sudden trouble walking, dizziness, loss of balance, or loss of coordination.
- Sudden headache or dizziness, for no obvious reason.

Notice the word that all those symptoms have in common, "Sudden". Almost all authorities advise us to look for "sudden" symptoms. But what if the symptoms are not sudden? My own symptoms seemed relatively slow to develop. They developed over a period of several days. For about two days, my balance slowly deteriorated, until I began to have obvious difficulties walking. Since I didn't have good balance to begin with, it took a while before it dawned on me that something new or different was happening.

And then, two days after I was admitted into a hospital, the muscles on the right side of my face began to sag a little, I began to slur my words, and my right arm and leg began to became noticeably weaker than my left limbs. The only thing that was "sudden" was my surprise when the doctors finally confirmed that rather than suffering from a progressive neurological problem, I had experienced a stroke. But there was nothing sudden about my symptoms — they developed relatively slowly. Maybe we need to redefine the warning signs of stroke to remove the term "sudden".

Of course, most people who have a stroke with very severe symptoms do seem to fit the standard description. Their symptoms do seem to come on "suddenly". But obviously that's not always the case, otherwise there would be no such thing as a silent stroke. By definition, a "silent stroke" is one that the victim is unaware of at the time of the episode. According to the American Heart Association, 8 million to 11 million people have silent strokes each year. That's a lot of strokes, silent or otherwise. Silent strokes are far more common than what we tend to think of as a classic stroke (American Heart Association News, 2016, December 16).[1]

In fact, according to the results of a survey published in the American Heart Association News (2017, May 1), "A third of U.S. adults have had symptoms consistent with a mini-stroke, but nearly no one – only 3 percent – called 911 for help, a survey released Monday shows" (p. 1).[2] I find that reading that article is

1 American Heart Association News. (2016, December 16). 'Silent strokes' found accidentally need treatment, statement says.   Retrieved   from https://www.heart.org/en/news/2018/05/01/silent-strokes-found-accidentally-need-treatment-statement-says

2 American Heart Association News. (2017, May 1). Survey: 1 in 3 adults may have had warning stroke, but most didn't seek

rather insulting —it gives the impression that the association is belittling the collective judgment of victims of silent strokes. For me at least, it conveys the notion that the American Heart Association is callous enough to imply that victims of silent strokes simply don't care enough to bother to report silent strokes. It suggests that most people who have silent strokes choose to just ignore them, as if they have a choice.

I must be missing something here. I thought that the definition of a silent stroke was one that doesn't cause any of the usual stroke symptoms, and most importantly, the victim is left unaware that he or she has even had a stroke. So how could they choose to report a silent stroke?

Some authorities claim that a silent stroke involves an area of the brain that isn't critical, so damage to that part of the brain doesn't affect normal functioning. But that's short-sighted, and too simplistic. I maintain that if the patient doesn't detect that a stroke is occurring, then by golly, that's a silent stroke, whether some expert is willing to admit it, or not.

As a stroke victim myself, and also a silent stroke victim, in my opinion, the pretense of that article is very misleading. I can guarantee you that I never chose to ignore my silent stroke. But apparently the state of confusion created in my brain by the min-

---

help.   Retrieved   from https://www.heart.org/en/news/2018/05/01/survey-1-in-3-adults-may-have-had-warning-stroke-but-most-didnt-seek-help stroke caused me to completely overlook those symptoms. Whether the failure to recognize it as a stroke was due to confusion, or lack of severity of the symptoms, is a moot point. I wasn't aware that I was having the episode, whether we agree to call it a silent stroke or not. I discovered evidence of that silent stroke, only after I had a much more serious stroke, several months later. How could I choose to ignore it when I wasn't even aware of it? I wonder if that's true in most other cases, also.

Statistics show that those symptoms (of silent strokes) never appear, in the majority of cases. And in many other cases, the symptoms are so subtle, that they're misjudged by a brain that may be clouded by the effects of the stroke. Doctors know that stroke victims suffer from a deterioration of cognizance (awareness), memory, and the ability to think clearly. To add insult to injury, that article appears to accuse victims of silent strokes of being so cavalier that they don't even bother to report silent strokes (despite the fact that silent strokes are by definition, undetected). So why should they assume that a stroke victim will immediately notice subtle symptoms that even they (the doctors) often cannot detect without sophisticated testing equipment?

In my case, after I had my (not-silent) stroke and I went to the emergency room, the ER doctor ran a few simple tests and was going to send me home, despite the fact that my balance was so poor that I was quite clumsy But after I mentioned my previous history of neurological issues, he decided to keep me overnight, and ordered a brain MRI scan for the next morning. The scan showed that I had experienced a stroke. The ER team had failed to recognize my stroke initially, because apparently I wasn't showing enough classic symptoms for them to identify. This is a perfect example of my point that even medical professionals can overlook a silent stroke or a mini-stroke — only this one wasn't a mini-stroke. The symptoms were just slow to reveal themselves.

At the time, I wasn't aware of the silent stroke that I had earlier. A few weeks after I had my stroke, I was attempting to write a few checks to pay some bills. I wasn't having much luck, because my handwriting looked similar to a child's scrawl, and I couldn't read it, no mater how hard I tried to write clearly. I understood what I was trying to write, and the process seemed to be as normal as always, except that my hand was very weak and shaky. But my hand and fingers couldn't properly transfer my thoughts to the paper. Only illegible scribbling showed up on the paper.

Then I happened to open the check register on the wrong page, and I noticed that the handwritten records from about three months earlier, looked similar. The writing wasn't quite as bad, but it was very difficult to read, over about a two-week period. This meets the criteria of a mini-stroke that specifies temporary symptoms. Why didn't I notice the handwriting problem when I was originally writing those records?

Thinking back, I could recall driving to an awards banquet one night at about the time when that two-week period began. I remember feeling confused, and even though it was a simple route that was easy to follow, and I had a GPS navigation device, I got lost, and I had a lot of trouble finding the site of the banquet. Obviously I must have had a silent stroke — and if I hadn't stumbled onto those check register entries, I never would have become aware of it. I wonder if I've had any other silent strokes.

Here's what happened when I had my actual stroke, about three months after that silent stroke. I got up one morning in the spring of 2017, ate breakfast, and proceeded to go about my day. Everything seemed normal, except that I was slightly clumsier than usual. That didn't concern me, because I'm a senior citizen (OK, I'm an old codger), with a pre-existing balance issue, and I'm often clumsier before I have my morning coffee. Otherwise, I felt fine. If there were other symptoms, I didn't notice them.

I have a brother who lives less than a half-mile away, and we often get together after noon, out in his tree-shaded yard, to discuss current events, and whatever else might come to mind. It provides a nice break in our schedules, and an opportunity to get in a little relaxation in the middle of the day. When I mentioned to him that my balance seemed to be worse than normal, he said that he had a similar problem the day before. He blamed it on a virus that was going around. To me, at the time, that sounded like a plausible explanation, so I didn't pursue it any further.

The next day, my balance was no better, and I didn't appear to have a virus. Later that afternoon, my balance seemed to be worse, so I asked my brother if he had time to take me to the emergency room at the local hospital to have it checked out. Naturally, he agreed.

After the ER team received the results of an EKG, and a few blood tests, they told us that everything appeared fine. They seemed to be ready to sent me back home, until I mentioned my history of neurological issues.

Back in 2009, one hot July morning, I noticed that my right hand was numb when I woke up. Since it wasn't unusual for one of my hands to fall asleep during the night, I naturally assumed that it would promptly wake up after I got up and started using it. But it didn't wake up. Instead, the numbness began to spread up my arm. I dug out some aspirin and took one. By then my arm was numb up to my elbow. By the time I got my shirt on, my arm was numb up to my shoulder. I took another aspirin, quickly finished dressing, and headed out the door to the car.

I intended to drive to my brother's house to see if he could take me to the ER. But he's a Realtor, and sometimes he has an early appointment, or he has to drive a long way to meet someone. Apparently this was one of those days, because when I got to his place, I could see that he was already gone. Rather than stop and call an ambulance, and then sit and wait for them, I made a quick decision to just keep driving. I was way out in the country, so it would take them at least 20 or 30 minutes to make the trip, if they left immediately. I could be at the hospital by then, if I kept driving (assuming that I was able to keep driving). So I kept driving.

About every 5 or 10 minutes, I would test the strength of my arm, and recall certain facts from memory, to verify that I was still capable of driving. My abilities seemed to continue to be normal. I stopped checking when I could see the hospital, just a few blocks away. By then, the entire right side of my face was also numb.

When I walked into the ER, they quickly escorted me to a small examination room and began hooking up monitors. My blood pressure and heart rate were high, naturally, since I assumed that I was having a stroke. But other than that, everything checked out fine. After the ER doctor reviewed all the test results, and my physical condition (no paralysis or loss of strength), he couldn't pinpoint the problem, so he called it a transient ischemic attack (TIA), and sent me home.

The next day, at the suggestion of a friend who is a pediatrician, I made an appointment with a neurologist, who proceeded to order many more tests (including a brain MRI). But those results were normal also, so he couldn't determine whether or not I actually had a mini-stroke. He did, however, based on my current neurological symptoms, diagnose me with Parkinson's disease. He based his diagnosis on my balance issues, abnormalities in my gait, a lack of normal knee and ankle reflexes, poor sense of feeling in my feet, and the fact that when I walked, my left arm swung back and forth normally, and the right one did not — it only moved through a small arc. Together, virtually all of those symptoms are characteristic of peripheral neuropathy, which I already knew I had. But I didn't believe that I had Parkinson's disease.

About 10 years earlier, in 1999, I had developed microscopic colitis (MC), which is an inflammatory bowel disease (IBD). For several months, I thought that I was just having relapses of the flu about once a month. But as the diarrhea episodes became more frequent, I decided that I must be the unluckiest guy around to be getting food poisoning so often. Eventually, when the diarrhea wouldn't stop, in early 2000, I had to admit that something much more ominous was going on.

Microscopic colitis causes severe nutrient malabsorption problems, so it's notorious for depleting vitamin D, magnesium, and after a few years, many of the "B" vitamins. The liver can store enough vitamin B-12 to last up to five years. But when B-12 becomes deficient, we run the risk of neurological damage. Vitamin D is the "fuel" on which our immune system operates. With a crippled immune system, we can't effectively fight off diseases and infections. The immune system is responsible for healing any damaged cells in the body. So with a compromised immune system, healing is slow, or it may be almost entirely prevented in some cases. The body cannot use the vitamins in the food we eat, or the supplements we take, until it converts them into the active forms, by a chemical process known as methylation.

Magnesium is required in order to complete many of these methylation actions, and various other essential chemical processes in the body — over 300 in all. And a deficiency of B-12 (cobalamin), B-5 (pantothenic acid), B-6 (pyridoxine), or B-9 (folate or folic acid) will eventually lead to neurological problems.

And note that despite the fact that the terms "folate" and "folic acid" are used interchangeably by almost everyone, they are not the same thing. Folate is a form of vitamin B-9 that occurs naturally. Most supplements, and enriched foods contain folic acid. The digestive system normally converts folate into the active form, 5-methyltetrahydrofolate (5-MTHF). But most folic acid has to be converted to the active form in the liver or other tissues, and this is a relatively slow and inefficient process. The process is so slow that un-metabolized folic acid tends to build up in the bloodstream, which may cause health issues (Tam, O'Connor, & Koren, 2012; Wiens & DeSoto, 2017; Harvard Heart Letter, 2008).[3, 4, 5]

I didn't learn this until it was too late, and so I suffered the consequences. I developed balance issues, and peripheral

---

3 Tam, C., O'Connor, D., & Koren, G. (2012,). Circulating unmetabolized folic acid: Relationship to folate status and effect of supplementation. Obstetrics and Gynecology International, 2012(485179) Retrieved from https://www.hindawi.com/journals/ogi/2012/485179/

4 Wiens, D. & DeSoto, M. C. (2017). Is high folic acid intake a risk factor for autism?—A review. Brain Sciences, 7(11), 149. Retrieved   from https://www.ncbi.nlm.nih.gov/pmc/articles/PMC5704156/

5 Harvard Heart Letter. (2008, December). Folic acid: Too much of a good thing? Retrieved from https://www.health.harvard.edu/newsletter_article/Folic_acid_Too_much_of_a_good_thing

neuropathy in my feet, because of deficiencies of magnesium, vitamin D, and several of the "B" vitamins. So my balance left a lot to be desired, several years before I had the TIAs, and long before I had the stroke.

Whenever we first notice symptoms, we automatically look for a reason. If we find one, it's human nature to assign undue relevance to it. In other words, we tend to decide that it's probably the reason for the symptoms, despite the fact that we have no proof. At any rate, my existing balance issues provided a reason (excuse) for me to overlook (or underestimate) the worsened balance issues that initially came with my stroke.

So because of my past history with neurological issues, they decided to keep me overnight in the hospital and do a brain scan the next morning. Sure enough, the scan revealed a narrowing in the fork of a small artery at the back of my brain, and an area of damaged brain tissue — an ischemic stroke. It was located in that part of the brain that controls memory, cognizance, balance, and coordination.

But here's something that I find puzzling. Even though my balance had deteriorated for almost two days before I checked into the ER, there was no significant difference between the strength of my right and left arms when the doctor tested them. At least neither I nor the doctor could detect any difference. Nor was there any noticeable difference in the strength of my legs. There were no other ordinary physical markers of a stroke, either, other than the worsened balance. Yet on the second day in the hospital, my right-sided weakness began to show up when a neurologist retested my arm and leg strength. And the right side of my face began to sag. A pattern of delayed symptoms such as this is said to be consistent with a mini-stroke, or TIA. And according to conventional wisdom, the symptoms should only be temporary.

I consider "temporary" to mean a few hours, to a few days at most. Yet my symptoms were noticeably worse two or three weeks later, than they were when I left the hospital. True, I slowly recovered most of my abilities by relearning how to do them, but I didn't recover automatically. I had to relearn how to do almost every task. And I still had obvious stroke symptoms, over two years after the stroke.

Back when I had the TIAs, the only symptom was paresthesia (numbness). The right side of my body became completely numb. The split even went right down the middle of my tongue. The ability to taste and sense the temperature of foods and liquids was completely absent in the right side of my mouth. It remained normal in the left side. I had to be careful that I didn't accidentally burn my mouth when eating.

There were no other symptoms, so they didn't keep me at the hospital much longer than the time it took to get the preliminary test results, and process the discharge papers. With the first TIA, the numbness lasted less than a day, and then began to fade away relatively quickly. When I had the second TIA (in May of 2010, which was about ten months later), most of the numbness faded away in less than a day, as before. But the numbness at the right side of my lips lingered, and slowly faded over several months.

However, when I had the stroke, there was no numbness, nor was there any tingling. In retrospect, I wonder if the TIAs were even related to the stroke, or if they were completely unrelated neurological events. At any rate, by the afternoon of the second day (after I was admitted into the hospital), my right leg had become so weak, and my balance so poor, that standing, without a walker, had become difficult. All my limbs were much weaker, but the right-sidedness of the stroke had become very evident.

A couple of physical therapists came by that afternoon and took me for a short walk down the hall. I suppose that verified, for the record, that I could walk with the aid of a walker, so when my doctor came by later, he informed me that I would probably be discharged the next morning before noon. But he scheduled one more test for me during the morning, an ultrasound scan (echocardiogram) of my heart.

Those results were satisfactory, so about noon, I was discharged. I found out later from a friend who's a physical therapist why they seemed to be in a rush to discharge me. She told me that the medicare treatment regulations specify that if a stroke victim is discharged within three days, the hospital doesn't have to provide that patient with physical therapy. And they receive bonus points that are added up at the end of the year to determine bonus payments from the government for reducing medicare expenses.

Stroke Recovery

The physical therapists had left a new walker for me in the hospital room, with instructions to take it home and use it. I had plenty of time to mull that over as I was getting dressed to go home, because it took me a long time to get dressed. When the time came to leave, I left the walker in the room, because I had decided that I would probably recover faster if I forced myself to walk without it. I was afraid that if I relied on a walker, I might never be able to get away from it.

In hindsight, that was clearly a poor decision, because getting around for the first few weeks without a walker was hell,. And I had the bruises to prove it. My leg strength, especially my right leg strength, seemed to continue to decline for the first two or three weeks, making walking extremely difficult. Apparently the stroke adversely affected my ability to make good decisions, because leaving the walker in the hospital room wasn't the only poor decision I made. I seemed to make poor decisions in general much more often after the stroke. At any rate, I walked out of that hospital on my own that day, by leaning on the rails whenever I needed extra support. I always wondered why hospitals were full of handrails. Now I know why. But I certainly didn't expect my leg strength (especially my right leg strength) to continue to deteriorate for two or three weeks after I left the hospital. Why didn't someone at the hospital warn me about that before I was discharged?

I never cease to be amazed by how inconsiderate the pharmaceu-tical industry appears to be. Surely they're well aware that stroke victims are very shaky and clumsy. One would think that they would make some effort to accommodate those needs. Yet they continue to dispense tiny pills commonly prescribed for stroke victims in containers that are difficult for the users to open and remove just one pill without spilling half of them. But then, I suppose those industry giants didn't get rich by worrying about stroke patients, or any other customers, for that matter.

And then there's the frequent problem with the inactive ingredients in prescription medications. Many of us have food allergies or food sensitivities, and far too many medications are formulated with ingredients that our bodies can't tolerate. Vitamin supplements have the same problem. Research shows that vitamins provide no benefits for people who have normal digestive systems and normal diets.

But for those of us who actually need vitamins, because of restricted diets, or compromised digestion, vitamin supplements can boost our health, and prevent disease. So why would the pharmaceutical companies manufacture vitamins that contain inactive ingredients that so many of the very customers who actually need those vitamins, can't tolerate? Apparently, they simply don't care.

This is especially important as we age, because our digestion becomes less efficient. In that situation, vitamin supplements can literally become life-savers, and they can add years to our lives, by helping to prevent disease. And those added years will come with significantly improved quality of life, due to improved health. Yet if you look at the labels of vitamin supplements, far too many of them contain unnecessary ingredients. Ingredients that don't need to be in there, and shouldn't be in there. Fortunately, some manufacturers have begun to recognize this problem, and more and more pharmaceutical products are being manufactured without those unnecessary ingredients. So check the labels carefully, before you buy, if you have any food sensitivities.

Here's an observation that I find interesting: When I was diagnosed with Parkinson's disease, one of the major diagnostic criteria that qualified me for a diagnosis was gait irregularities. Part of that criteria is the hand swinging pattern as a patient walks. When a normal person walks, they swing their arms in sync with their opposite legs. In other words, as they step forward with their right leg, they also swing their left arm forward. And as they step forward with their left leg, so that their right leg falls behind, their right arm swings forward in sync with the left leg, and their left arm swings back in sync with their right leg. And the pattern repeats with each step. The amplitude of the arcs through which the arms swing is normally proportional to (slightly less than) or roughly equal to the arcs described by the legs, and it's uniform on both sides.

Before the stroke, my left arm swung normally. But the arc through which my right arm sung (both fore and aft) was very limited. The total arc through which my right arm swung appeared to be about one-fourth to one-third of normal. Furthermore, as I was walking, I landed on the balls of my feet, rather than on my heels, like a normal person. In other words, the initial contact of each foot as it landed on the floor, was on the ball of the foot, instead of the heel.

But this is how a bowhunter moves forward when they're stalking game, and I was a bowhunter at the time. So was this abnormality due to an unintentional habit formed-during years of bowhunting, or was it due to the nerve damage that causes peripheral neuropathy?

Regardless of the reason, a few months after my stroke, I was surprised to notice that as my walking ability began to improve, my gait seemed to be normal again, and my hand-swinging pattern appeared to be normal. When I walked, my feet landed on their heels, just as they should. Obviously, most of the nerve paths previously used by my brain to deliver instructions to my leg and arm muscles as I walked, had been destroyed. So my brain was forced to find new pathways to deliver those instructions. Clearly, those alternate pathways were not destroyed or damaged by the stroke, because I was never totally unable to walk. If all of the nerve pathways had been blocked, I wouldn't have been able to walk at all.

I find the fact that the same instructions delivered by the brain using an alternate network of nerves somehow corrected my previously corrupted gait to be extremely fascinating. It makes me wonder just where the corruption originally existed. Maybe I've been searching in all the wrong places, but I've never heard of a pre-existing neurological problem that was corrected by a stroke. Based on available information, I assumed that strokes only cause problems.

In my case, the net result of my stroke was to leave me much weaker and clumsier overall, and the strength and coordination of my right arm and leg were diminished to a much greater extent. But my right side limbs were not completely disabled (thank goodness), and I could still walk, with considerable difficulty. If I lost any past memories, I'm not aware of that, although my short term memory was rather poor after the stroke, and it didn't seem to improve by any noticeable amount as I recovered. My cognizance was definitely worse. I tended to become confused, and I tried to do many things (such as tightening or loosening a nut on a bolt) backwards after the stroke. As far as dexterity and coordination are concerned, I remembered how to do virtually everything, I just couldn't get my hands or feet to do them automatically.

Consequently, I had to relearn how to walk, eat, shave, comb my hair, put on my clothes, drive, type on a keyboard, use a computer mouse, and virtually everything else that we learn to do automatically as we grow up. I relearned how to do most things well enough to get by within a few months. But I was far from being symptom-free.

After over two years of recovery, I seemed to have reached a point where I could no longer detect any improvement progress. I was much better, but I was still slower, clumsier, and made many more mistakes than I did before the stroke. Perhaps this was as good as I could expect to get. After all, I had come a long way, and I could certainly live with this level of performance and quality of life. As we say in engineering, it's close enough for most practical purposes. So all-in-all, I was happy with my recovery, and thankful that I had been able to come this far. But still, I longed to be better, if that were possible.

Chapter 2

The Discovery That Kick-Started My Stalled Stroke Recovery

One of the attributes that you develop in engineering is the nagging desire to find a better way to do things, whether you're analyzing a design or a process. When you're trying to solve a very difficult problem, and you've tried all the conventional methods without success, what do you do? You think outside the box, of course. In this case, that means looking past the conventional treatment methods. It means looking everywhere and anywhere for clues that might lead to a better solution.

Looking back, if I had known when I had the stroke, what I know now, I would have begun taking magnesium threonate immediately. But I was unaware of the product. For my treatment, my doctors only recommended that I take Plavix (which I was already taking before the stroke, due to the TIAs) and a statin. I also take a small dose of lisinopril (10 mg) to reduce my blood pressure. But I was already taking that before the stroke, also (I started taking it after the second TIA), and I didn't have a hypertension problem to begin with. The lisinopril was simply a precaution to push my blood pressure below normal. I check my blood pressure every morning before I take any medications, and if the systolic pressure is below 100 mmHG, I skip the lisino-pril.

But no medical professional, nor anyone else, suggested (or even mentioned) magnesium threonate. I stumbled upon it acciden-tally, while reviewing recent research involving magnesium (for a different project). I discovered it and started learning more about it, more than two years after my stroke.

I certainly don't blame my doctors for not telling me about magnesium threonate. They may have been aware of it, but they couldn't justify recommending it. They're hostages of an overly-zealous legal system. If a doctor recommends a treatment that's not endorsed and accepted by the medical community in general, and anything goes wrong with the treatment, they will surely be the target of a lawsuit that threatens their reputation and career, to say nothing of the loss to their bank account. Their insurance rates may go up to unrealistic levels, and they may even lose the ability to buy insurance. So the very real threat of legal action severely limits the likelihood that most doctors will recommend an unapproved treatment to a patient.

The research article that I came across was based on data from the results of a trial published in the Journal of Alzheimer's Disease in 2016 (Liu, Weinger, Lu, Xue, & Sadeghpour, 2016).[6] It

---

6 Liu, G., Weinger, J. G., Lu, Z.-L., Xue, F. & Sadeghpour, S. (2016). Efficacy and safety of MMFS-01, a synapse density enhancer, for treating cognitive impairment in older adults: A randomized, double-blind, placebo-controlled trial. Journal of Alzheimer's Disease, 49(4), 971-990. Retrieved from https://www.ncbi.nlm.nih.gov/pmc/articles/PMC4927823/

was only a small study, so normally, I wouldn't have paid much attention to the claims made by the authors. But the fact that the study was done with so much care to insure the integrity of the data, caught my attention. It was conducted as a randomized, double-blind, placebo-controlled trial — about as good as it gets with medical research. Published research proves that most of the claims made by medical researchers are false (Ioannidis, J. P.A., 2005).[7] Bogus medical articles abound, unfortunately. Sometimes,you have to interpret the data yourself, in order to get an accurate picture of the research. But false conclusions are far less likely with randomized, double-blind, placebo-controlled trials.

According to the claims made about magnesium threonate, it has a very impressive ability to improve memory and cognitive function. And the data appear to back that up. In the trial, magnesium threonate was shown to be capable of rolling back the brain functioning of older adults by an average of ten years of age. Furthermore, the data showed that magnesium threonate achieved these results by increasing the number of synapses in the brain.

Synapses are special nerve receptors that allow the transmission of nerve signals across gaps (between neurons), at the ends of nerve fibers. In other words, when our brain generates an electrical signal to search for a memory stored somewhere in our brain, that signal has to cross many gaps (synapses) before it

---

7 Ioannidis, J. P.A. (2005). Why most published research findings are false. PLoS Medicine, 2(8), e124. Retrieved from https://www.ncbi.nlm.nih.gov/pmc/articles/PMC1182327/

reaches the correct nerve fiber that will lead it to the proper memory. There are neurons (nerve cells) on each side of the gap to send and receive these signals. And there are many paths available so that the signal can reach the target by many optional routes. But if the proper functioning of some of those synapses (or the neurons on either side) have been compromised , then those routes to the memory may be effectively blocked. If enough routes are blocked, then that particular memory (and possibly others) has become unavailable, and our brain will not be able to retrieve it.

Likewise, when our brain issues a command to instruct certain muscles to perform certain tasks, that signal has to travel through the central nervous system, passing through many nerve passageways, and across many synapses, in order to reach the proper target cells at the muscles. Because there are so many path options, if a few are blocked, we probably won't even notice. But, if enough of them are blocked (if enough neurons or synapses become disabled) we may lose control of that muscle.

During an ischemic stroke, it's claimed that approximately 14 billion synapses are destroyed per minute (Saver, 2006).[8] That's not the only damage caused by a stroke, obviously — huge numbers of neurons and nerve fibers are destroyed each minute, also. But I focused on the synapses, because magnesium threonate is promoted as a substance that will increase the number

---

8   Saver, J. L., (2006). Time is brain—Quantified. Stroke, 37 (1), 263–266.   Retrieved   from https://www.ahajournals.org/doi/10.1161/01.STR.0000196957.55928.ab

of synapses in the brain. And presumably. this capability also extends to the central nervous system .

Increasing synapses after a stroke is important, because this is one of the ways (along with increased neuron production) in which the body normally tries to recover after a stroke. Or at least this is how it attempts to recover. Sometimes there are issues that limit our ability to utilize this attempted restoration process.

It seemed to be a relatively safe product, so I decided to try it. I was already taking a magnesium supplement (I had been taking it for years, even before the stroke), so I adjusted my dose, to allow for the extra magnesium in the magnesium threonate. The labeled dose of the brand of magnesium threonate that I selected is three capsules daily. The total amount of elemental magnesium contained in three capsules is listed as 147 milligrams (mg), so I reduced my regular magnesium supplement by 100 mg. Since this is a relatively new product, just to be on the safe side, I started my treatment with one capsule per day for a few days to make sure that I didn't have any adverse reactions to it before increasing the dose to two capsules per day for a few days. Since there were no adverse reactions within a week, I boosted the dose to three capsules per day. After about three or four weeks I began to notice improvements in my memory and cognizance.

Remember, though, that personal observations such as this are subject to personal bias and misinterpretation, so we need to be very careful in how much confidence we place in them. Also, because of my age, (78, as of this writing) we have to be careful that we don't confuse common symptoms that arise due to advancing age with symptoms caused by stroke.

It's well-known that balance, coordination, cognizance, and memory normally diminish with increasing age. This was previously blamed on age-related decreases in neurons. But more recent research shows that while some neurons are indeed lost due to aging, the number of neurons lost is actually a relatively small percentage, on the order of 2–4 % (Jarrett, 2017,).[9] Obviously this small amount doesn't explain why so many of us experience significant neurological loses as we age. Researchers have not been able to pinpoint the exact reason why this happens. My own opinion is that the loss of plasticity in the brain is the main cause of age-related loss of abilities. Brain plasticity (which is defined in the next chapter) refers to the ability of the brain to change continuously throughout an individual's life. The loss of plasticity surely results in damage to neurons, synapses, nerve fibers, and other components of our complex neurological systems, over time.

As a sidelight, I note that many (perhaps most) symptoms that most doctors attribute to advanced age are actually due to issues caused by diet (food sensitivities), long-term vitamin or mineral deficiencies, or the side effects of medications. Many of us have been in a situation where our doctor asks us if we have any aches or pains, and when we admit that we have, and then

---

9   Jarrett, C. (2017, December 1). "Significant loss of neurons is a normal part of ageing" and other brain cell myths. Research Digest -The British Psycological Society. Retrieved from https://digest.bp-s.org.uk/2017/12/01/significant-loss-of-neurons-is-a-normal-part-of-ageing-and-other-brain-cell-myths/

proceed to describe the symptoms, she or he simply dismisses those symptom by attributing them to "old age", as if that somehow makes the symptoms "normal", and OK to trivialize. In most cases the actual cause can be discovered if we really want to resolve those symptoms, and that cause is virtually never simply "old age".

Food sensitivities are becoming more common these days. And the older we get, the more likely we are to become deficient in certain vitamins and minerals, especially if we have to eat a restricted diet because of food sensitivities, or for any other reason.

Side effects caused by drugs, and interactions with other drugs are common. Because their livelihood depends on writing prescriptions in order to resolve medical problems, most doctors tend to underestimate the problems caused by drug side effects, and interactions with other drugs.. But in fact, prescription medications are a common cause of symptoms in older people (Ruscin & Sunny, 2018).[10] Remember that older individuals tend to take far more medications than younger people Often, two or more of those medications may have known adverse interactions that our doctor may overlook. In general, our pharmacist is much more likely to spot potential drug interaction problems than our doctors. So it's a very good idea to ask our pharmacist

---

10 Ruscin, J. M., & Sunny, A. L., (2018, December). Drug-related problems in older adults. Retrieved from https://www.merckmanuals.com/professional/geriatrics/drug-therapy-in-older-adults/drug-related-problems-in-older-adults

about possible problems with our other medications when filling a prescription for the first time.

And even in cases where the doctor correctly attributes a symptom to a prescribed medication, rather than to advise the patient to stop using that medication, the doctor will often write a prescription for another medication to counteract the side effects of the first medication. And often that medication will cause additional side effects. The patient is caught in a cruel cycle, and eventually they will usually just give up and tolerate the side effects, if they're not intolerable.

But in many cases, drug side effects may not show up until after a patient has been using a medication for a long time. In that situation, neither the doctor nor the patient is likely to attribute the symptoms to any of the medications involved. And over the years, as we get older, and accumulate prescriptions, the list of symptoms from unrecognized causes can slowly grow. The point is, as we grow older, we shouldn't automatically assume that any of our symptoms are due to "old age", even when our doctors are naive enough to suggest that they are.

Getting back to the main subject of this discussion, another caveat that we have to be aware of when we try to interpret personal experiences is the placebo effect (National Center for Complementary and Integrative Health. (2017).[11] The placebo effect can be far more powerful than most people realize (Brynie,

---

11 National Center for Complementary and Integrative Health. (2017). Placebo effect. Retrieved from https://nccih.nih.gov/health/placebo

2012, January 10).[12] With all that in mind, some of my personal observations after taking magnesium threonate for a while are listed below.

After taking magnesium threonate for three or four weeks, I found that my ability to recall names and events was noticeably improved. I was able to recall most names within a few seconds. Previously, it often took me several hours to half-a-day to recall them. Sure, I still come up empty-handed once in a while. Who doesn't? But that happens a lot less often now.

After a few weeks of treatment, I could focus my thoughts better, so that I could make better decisions. I made fewer bad decisions, and fewer mistakes. At that point, I still hadn't noticed any improvement in my balance, or coordination, or any other lingering stroke symptoms. That was discouraging, but I continued the treatment.

Prior to starting the treatment, it usually took a while to get to sleep after going to bed, and I had been waking up at least two or three times during the night, needing to use the bathroom. After returning to bed, getting back to sleep usually took longer than it should have.

After taking the magnesium threonate for several weeks, I found that I seldom woke up more than once during the night, needing to use the bathroom. And afterward, getting back to sleep was

12 Brynie, F., (2012, January 10). The placebo effect: How it works. Retrieved from https://www.psychologytoday.com/us/blog/brain-sense/201201/the-placebo-effect-how-it-works

usually easier. On some nights, I slept right through until my usual time for getting up (about an hour before sunup). This has a lot of advantages for a stroke victim, because better sleep means improved healing and alertness, which translates to better balance and coordination. And theoretically, sleeping better should result in a lower average blood pressure, which could reduce the odds of having another stroke in the future.

After taking it longer (for a couple of months, or more), I find that on some nights, my brain seems to be more active. It seems to be more easily stimulated, and if I wake up, I have difficulty getting back to sleep, due to concentrating on a book I'm writing, or something else. But since this happened occasionally well before the stroke, maybe I'm just experiencing a return to a more normal level (for me, at least), pattern of brain activity. All-in-all, I believe that on the average, I'm sleeping better, and deriving more benefit from my sleep.

Since I take my blood pressure every morning, I was able to monitor the blood pressure issue. For a few weeks, lower blood pressure seemed to be the norm, but as time went on, according to my records,I can't say that my average blood pressure has been any lower in the long run. If anything, it's sometimes somewhat more erratic, probably due to how well I sleep on any particular night. My brain seems to be more productive now, making writing easier, because it's easier to keep track of ideas and thoughts.

I've always been clumsier when I was sleepy. I assume that applies to everyone. But the stroke seemed to magnify that effect. After the stroke, when I first got out of bed in the morning, or any time that I wasn't fully alert, I tended to be noticeably clumsier than at other times, due to poor balance. And as I would expect, my balance was significantly improved after drinking my first cup of coffee in the morning, to boost my alertness. After taking magnesium threonate for about six weeks, though, my balance was noticeably improved when I was drowsy. I wasn't nearly as clumsy.

Some of that improvement (maybe all of it) is probably due to better sleep. The research article also mentioned that subjects in the trial reported improved sleep. That certainly doesn't detract from the treatment, though. I'll take improvements any way I can get them.

Whatever the reason, after taking magnesium threonate for about twelve weeks, even when I got out of bed in the middle of the night, most of the clumsiness that was previously caused by drowsiness seemed to be gone. My balance was surprisingly steady early in the morning. That's a very impressive improvement, to say the least. I wouldn't call this product a miracle cure, but do any medications actually fall into that category? I haven't encountered any, but there may be some that qualify in specific situations.

All-in-all, I believe I can honestly say that my balance when I'm drowsy is equal to or better now, than at any other time in my life. That's not true for when I'm fully alert, of course (my balance was much better when I was younger). But the improvement is quite noticeable when I'm sleepy, especially in the wee hours of the morning. I no longer worry nearly as much about falling when I get up during the night to use the bathroom. That's very important, because falls are probably the main cause of loss of mobility for senior citizens. That said, I'm still cautious when I get up during the night, because I'm aware of far too many older friends who never were able to recover from their first serious fall.

My balance and coordination in general are significantly improved. I've noticed that whenever I'm working around machinery and heavy equipment, and I have to duck under or step over something, it's much easier to do now. Before, I was clumsier, and If I had to both step over and duck under something at the same time, I had to grab onto some support to keep from losing my balance and falling. Now, I don't need any extra support.

After the stroke, I always had to lean on something for support whenever I was putting on or taking off my shorts. I often tried to do that without any support, but I was never able to come even close to being successful. After eleven or twelve weeks of taking magnesium threonate, I found that my balance was improved enough that I was able to put on or take off my shorts without leaning against or holding onto any support. I'm not sure if I'll ever be able to put on or take off my Levis without any support, but I'm optimistic that I may be able to do that eventually. Just being able to put on my shorts without having to lean against something for support was more improvement than I expected.

The Discovery That Kick-Started My Stalled Stroke Recovery

I've noticed an improvement in my ability to accurately click on small targets on a computer screen with a mouse, also. Right after the stroke, I was as wild as the wind when I tried to click on those targets. It usually took me many attempts before I succeeded. Of course I slowly improved as I recovered. But I finally reached a point where I wasn't improving any more. Magnesium threonate got me past that point, and I'm improving again. Now I can accurately click on those targets almost as fast as I could before the stroke.

My stroke occurred slightly more than two-and-a-half years ago (as of this writing), and I've been taking magnesium threonate about four months. I'll admit right up front that I'm clumsier these days than I was as a young man, I'm not as well coordi- nated, and I'm slower than I was decades ago. But probably that's mostly because I'm an old codger now. So I surely walk like an old man, and my reduced coordination shows my age. But I no longer walk like an old man who's had a stroke, and I'm not as fumble-fingered as I was, thanks to magnesium threonate. You would have to observe me for a long time to detect that I've had a stroke —it's no longer obvious, like it was before I started taking the product. My gait is better than it was fifteen or twenty years ago.

Before I started taking magnesium threonate, I had managed to climb about six or eight feet up a ladder in order to perform a few simple maintenance tasks. But I was afraid to attempt climbing higher, because I was still too weak and shaky, and I didn't trust my balance. If you've had a stroke, you know what I mean.

Stroke Recovery

After taking magnesium threonate for about twelve weeks, I had enough confidence to be able to climb about twice that high in order to get up on a roof and repair a minor problem with my TV antenna rotor. That was something that I had previously assumed I would never be able to do again.

A stroke definitely changes our lives, and some of the changes are drastic and very unpleasant. But in my case at least, I have to say that surprisingly, not all of the changes were negative. I find that my perceptiveness, and appreciation of the little things in life have increased. I find it much easier to focus on the good things around me. The bad things are easier to correct, and if I can't correct them, they're easier to ignore.

It seems that virtually everything used to treat health issues comes with a few unpleasant effects, as well. Many prescription medications are known to have serious side effects for some people. Alas, I discovered that magnesium threonate may also have a few caveats. I mentioned a few pages back that some nights it seems to make my mind more active, making getting to sleep more difficult. After I had taken magnesium threonate for about fourteen weeks, I developed a tooth infection, and needed to take an antibiotic. I chose Cipro, because it's the only antibiotic that never triggers a microscopic colitis flare. And despite all the dire black box warnings on the label, it has never caused any side effect symptoms for me.

When I started taking the antibiotic, the first night I had significant trouble sleeping. I attributed that to the pain, because the infection was quite painful. But the second night, I got absolutely no sleep at all. My mind continuously churned with confused thoughts that completely prevented me from getting to sleep. I finally gave up and got up about eight o'clock, dog-tired, as the saying goes.

I'm 78, and during my lifetime I've stayed up all night on at least three or four occasions, so I didn't get any sleep on those nights. Back before I figured out how to resolve my microscopic colitis symptoms (that I previously mentioned), I was so sick and achy and bloated (due to undiscovered food sensitivities that were perpetuating the symptoms) that on many nights, sleep was very difficult. But I always managed to get at least a few hours of sleep, anyway.

This was the first time in my 78 years that I spent a sleepless night in bed. I've taken Cipro many times before, without noticing any sleep problems. The tooth pain was not as severe the second night. Therefore I have to conclude that the magnesium threonate may have contributed to the sleepless night. It's certainly possible that it may have an undocumented drug interaction with Cipro, or even with antibiotics in general. After all, there hasn't been much actual medical research done on magnesium threonate. And there's not likely to be much science-based research done on it in the future, because of the fact that magnesium can't be patented, so there's little potential for huge profits to be made.

My blood pressure was elevated by at least thirty points that morning, at 142/80 mmHG, and my heart rate was 80 beats per minute (BPM), which is also high for me. While it's certainly possible that the infection might have caused the uptick, it's more likely that lack of sleep was almost entirely responsible, since the problem occurred on only that one morning. So I skipped taking the magnesium threonate the next day. Sure enough, the following night I slept much better. I had a little difficulty initially getting to sleep, but this could have been due to apprehension. After I had slept for a couple of hours, I was awakened by a small thunderstorm. I had no trouble getting back to sleep afterward. My blood pressure that morning was 109/71, with a heart rate of 70. These are much more typical numbers for me. So I decided to continue to postpone taking any more magnesium threonate for the duration of the seven-day antibiotic treatment.

If I had any loss of balance, coordination, or any other ability during the first day, I didn't notice. I did notice however, that after I took a shower before going to bed, I was unable to put on my shorts without losing my balance. I had to lean against something. That didn't concern me, because it might have just been a coincidence. That night I slept even better. But when I got up to start the day, it didn't take long to notice that my balance and coordination seemed to have deteriorated slightly. By the third morning, there was no question that my balance and coordination was declining. After a week, I seemed to be back to about where I was before I started taking the magnesium threonate.

That answered a question I had about how long we need to take magnesium threonate. Apparently it needs to be taken indefinitely in order to maintain any gains. But even though I'm now aware of that, I would still discontinue taking magnesium threonate during a treatment with Cipro, because I consider good sleep to be paramount.

When I resumed taking the magnesium threonate after finishing the Cipro treatment, it seemed to take only a few days to regain most of the progress that I had made previously by taking the magnesium threonate. To illustrate this, by the third day, I was able to put on or take off my shorts again, without losing my balance.

That was my experience with magnesium threonate — yours might be somewhat different. You can decide for yourself whether you feel that a treatment is worth a try. Obviously, I can't guarantee that it will help you in your stroke recovery, but it certainly helped me. It takes a while to get results — it seems to take a few weeks or more to begin to show any benefits. But in my case at least, the improvements were better than I anticipated. I don't mean to convey the impression that magnesium threonate has completely reversed all the remaining symptoms of my stroke. It hasn't. That would be too good to be true, considering the broad extent of the damage done by the stroke to so many neurological functions. I'm simply saying that it has significantly helped me to minimize the most persistent and troublesome symptoms of my stroke that remained after my recovery seemed to have stalled.

And the little experiment that I did by withholding the treatment for a week while I was taking an antibiotic, showed that the magnesium threonate was indeed responsible for the neurological function improvements. This was further supported when I resumed the treatment and the improvements were restored within a few days.

Eventually I decided that reducing the dose of my magnesium supplement when I began to take magnesium threonate was counterproductive. After a few months I began to develop the tell-tale symptoms of nocturnal leg and foot cramps, muscle aches, and fatigue, indicating that I was developing a chronic magnesium deficiency. So I restored my daily magnesium glycinate dose to 300 mg, and experienced almost instant relief from those symptoms. Therefore I have to conclude that virtually all of the elemental magnesium in magnesium threonate goes to the brain, and very little, if any, goes to other cells in the body. If that's the case, then obviously there's no need to adjust one's magnesium supplementation pattern when beginning to take magnesium threonate. So every day, I now take 300 mg of magnesium glycinate (3 tablets), and 147 mg of magnesium threonate (3 capsules), divided up between meals, and I continue to do well.

Magnesium threonate does not require a prescription. Based on my experience, it appears to be a low or no risk treatment option that can benefit not only older people with dementia or memory issues, but recovering stroke victims as well. I can't say that it totally eliminated all my remaining stroke issues, but it certainly helped, and overall, my memory and cognizance is significantly improved. As stroke victims, we all have the built-in ability to recover (or at least attempt to recover) from a stroke. Why not make the most of it?

Chapter 3

A Few Thoughts About Post-Stroke Depression

Post-stroke depression is common, and it's often a very serious problem. It usually surfaces about two weeks after the stroke. Since post-stroke depression can have such a devastating effect on anyone's recovery, it's an issue that should not be ignored. Outside of the obvious depressive situation due to the loss of capabilities in general, exactly what causes the high rates of post-stroke depression is unclear.

Research suggests that as the body attempts to regenerate neurons to replace those destroyed by the stroke, mild chronic stress may trigger a chemical reaction that appears to restrict the plasticity of the newly generated neurons(Yu, Cheng, Ali, Wang, Le, Chibaatar, & Guo, 2019).[13] Brain plasticity (or neural plasticity, or neuroelasticity,) refers to the ability of the brain to change continuously throughout an individual's life in order to

---

13 Yu, D., Cheng, Z., Ali, A. I., Wang, J., Le, K., Chibaatar, E., & Guo, Y. (2019). Chronic unexpected mild stress destroys synaptic plasticity of neurons through a glutamate transporter, GLT-1, of astrocytes in the ischemic stroke rat. Neural Plasticity, 2019 (1615925). Retrieved from https://www.hindawi.com/journals/np/2019/1615925/abs/

accommodate changing circumstances. When neural plasticity is compromised, then neurological recovery after a stroke will surely be limited.

The actual mechanics of depression are still unknown (after all these years of study). But it's not just a matter of chemical imbalance in the brain, despite the fact that the chemical imbalance theory still lingers. What happens in the brain to cause depression appears to be far more complex than that. The Harvard Medical School website (2019, June 24) offers a good explanation (with regular updates) of current thoughts on the issue.[14] Attitude may be more important than anything else.

Personally, I had absolutely no issues with depression. That may have simply been due to good luck. Or it may have been due to the fact that I considered myself extremely lucky that the stroke was not worse. Strokes can always be worse, (unless they're fatal). I had no remorse. So I never dwelled on any negative thoughts about how unpleasant it was, and I never asked, "Why me?" I was just mighty glad that I was still alive and able to look forward to getting better, so that some day I might be able to finish a book that I had started. In other words, I accidentally had the right attitude.

I certainly didn't enjoy it, but living with the stroke symptoms was so much better than not living, that I never looked back. I didn't blame myself, or anyone else, or anything that I had done,

---

14 Harvard Medical School. (2019, June 24). What causes depression? Retrieved from https://www.health.harvard.edu/mind-and-mood/what-causes-depression

so I had no regrets. But most of all, I knew that I would get better. That provided hope, and hope is the one thing that gives us incentive and allows us to tolerate virtually anything. Without hope, incentives are lost.

Early on, my doctors kept asking me if I had any suicidal thoughts. I couldn't understand the reason for that. Why on earth would I want to commit suicide? I thought they were out of touch with reality, until I read about the problem of post-stroke depression. Then I realized how lucky I was that I considered myself to be lucky, so that I had remained optimistic about my recovery. Apparently that kept me from developing the usual post-stroke depression.

So please don't allow stress to defeat your recovery. As indicated by the research I cited, the post-stroke depression caused by chronic unexpected mild stress can actually prevent your body from being able to recover normally. Do whatever you have to do in order to minimize stress, but make stress-control a priority.

Many people have good results with meditation, or yoga. Of course, yoga may not be an option after a stroke — at least not for a while. And it may never be an option for some of us. But we can always listen to music, or specially-prepared relaxation recordings, or simply sit outside and observe the beauty of nature and the wonders of the world around us.

Relaxing and doing whatever it takes to keep our thoughts positive and free of stress and worry takes much less effort than dwelling on negative thoughts. Entertaining negative thoughts

Stroke Recovery

can only have negative consequences, The net cost of negative thinking can be devastating — it can steal part, or possibly even most, of our stroke recovery. That can make a positive attitude, priceless.

Note that magnesium threonate is claimed to increase neural plasticity. Therefore, taking magnesium threonate might be expected to be somewhat protective of newly regenerated neurons and synapses, which should help to reduce the damage caused by stress and post-stroke depression. Just to be on the safe side, though, I firmly believe that we should do everything within reason to try to minimize stress. This is always a good idea, but it's critical to a good recovery from a stroke. So if you want to maximize your recovery gains, besides taking magnesium threonate, do whatever you have to do to relax and maintain a positive, optimistic frame of mind. This is one situation where attitude can make all the difference in the world.

About the Author

Wayne Persky BSME

Wayne Persky was born, grew up, and currently lives in Central Texas. He is a graduate of the University of Texas at Austin, College of Engineering, with postgraduate studies in mechanical engineering, mathematics, and computer science. He has teaching experience in engineering, and business experience in farming and agribusiness.

After the onset of severe digestive system issues and various other health problems in the late 1990s, he went through extensive clinical testing, but the gastroenterologist failed to discover the problem; microscopic colitis. After all the tests, not surprisingly, he was told by his gastroenterologist that there was nothing wrong with him.

Unable to find a medical solution, he was forced to use his research skills to resolve his health issues himself. After doing extensive on-line research, and studying various published medical research articles, he realized that he had microscopic colitis, and the symptoms were being perpetuated by the inflammation caused by food sensitivities.

It took a year and a half of trial and error diet experimentation, and careful record-keeping, to track down all of the food issues. But once he eliminated all of those foods from his diet, all of the symptoms stopped, and he got his health back. He founded and

Stroke Recovery

administrates an online microscopic colitis discussion and support forum, while continuing to live on a farm in Central Texas. In 2015 he founded the Microscopic Colitis Foundation, and he continues to serve as it's president and as a contributing author to the Foundation's Newsletter.

During the last week of March, in 2017, he had a stroke, and he began his recovery. Eventually, he was able to recover to the point where no residual symptoms were significant enough to be a problem.

Contact Details:

Wayne Persky can be contacted at:
Persky Farms
19242 Darrs Creek Rd
Bartlett, TX 76511
USA

Tel: 1(254)718-1125
Tel: 1(254)527-3682

Email: wayne@perskyfarms.com
Email: wayne@microscopiccolitisfoundation.org
Email: wayne@waynepersky.com

For information and support regarding microscopic colitis, visit:

http://www.microscopiccolitisfoundation.org/
To view or participate in the Microscopic Colitis Discussion and Support Forum, go to:

http://www.perskyfarms.com/phpBB2/index.php

Made in the USA
Monee, IL
05 November 2020

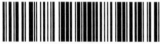
46790565R00031